The Ultimate Anti-Inflammatory Vegetarian Cookbook

A Vibrant Collection of Fully Vegetarian Recipes for your Healthy Meals

Natalie Worley

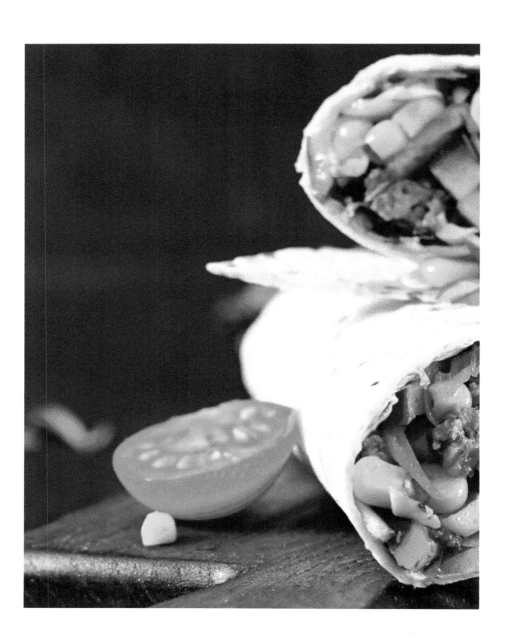

any techniques outlined in this book.

by reading this document, the reader agrees that under no circumstances is the author responsible for any losses, direct or indirect, which are incurred as a result of the use of information contained within this document, including, but not limited to, — errors, omissions, or inaccuracies.

Table of Contents

Burrito Zoodles

Prep Time: 25 min | **Cook Time:** 15 min | **Serve:** 4

- Coconut oil 2 T

- Onion 1 medium, chopped

- Garlic 2 cloves minced

- Chili powder 1 tsp.

- Cumin .5 tsp. ground

- Kosher salt as desired

- Black pepperas desired

- Black beans 15 oz. drained and rinsed

- Cherry tomatoes 1 c halved

- Red enchilada sauce 1 c

- Cheddar 1 c shredded

- Monterey Jack 1 c shredded

- Zoodles 14 oz.

1.Add the oil to the skillet before placing it on the stove over a burner turned to medium heat.

2.Add in the carrot and onion and allow both to cook approximately 5 minutes before adding in the garlic and allowing it to cook approximately 60 seconds.

3.Mix in the cumin, chili powder, salt, and pepper before adding in the cheese, enchilada sauce, cherry tomatoes, and black beans.

4.Allow everything to simmer approximately 10 minutes before adding in the zoodles and tossing to coat. Let the zoodles cook approximately 3 minutes, stirring regularly.

Red Pepper Zoodles

Prep Time: 10 min | **Cook Time:** 25 min | **Serve:** 4

- Red bell peppers 1

- Almond milk 1 c

- Coconut oil 1 T

- Salt 1 tsp.

- Garlic 1 clove

- Almond Coconut oil .25 c

1.Prepare a baking sheet by lining it with foil.

2.Add the bell peppers to the baking sheet before placing them on the top level of your broiler and letting them cook until blackened.

3.Once they have cooled you can remove the skins,

stems, seeds, and ribs.

4.Add the results, along with the remaining sauce
ingredients and blend thoroughly. Season as desired.

5.Serve with zoodles and a variety of potential toppings,
including truffle oil, goat cheese, parmesan cheese, or
parsley.

Zoodles Marinara

Prep Time: 15 min | **Cook Time:** 15 min | **Serve:** 4

- Extra virgin coconut oil 2 T

- White onions .5 c diced

- Garlic cloves 6 minced

- Tomatoes 14 oz. diced

- Tomato paste 2 T

- Basil leaves .5 c roughly-chopped loosely packed

- Coarse salt 5 tsp

- Black pepper .25 tsp

- Cayenne 1 pinch

- Zucchinis 2 large spiralized

- Parmesan cheese as desired

1.Add the oil to the skillet before placing it on the stove over a burner turned to a medium heat.

2.Add in the onion and allow it to cook approximately 5 minutes before adding in the garlic and allowing it to cook approximately 60 seconds.

3.Mix in the crushed red pepper flakes, pepper, salt, basil tomato paste, and tomatoes and combine thoroughly.

4.Allow the sauce to simmer before reducing the heat to medium/low. Let the sauce simmer an additional 15 minutes or until the oil takes on a deep orange color, which indicates the sauce is thickened and reduced. Season as desired.

5.Add in the zoodles and let them soften approximately 2 minutes.

6.Top with parmesan cheese before serving.

Zoodle Japchae

Prep Time: 15 min | **Cook Time:** 8 min | **Serve:** 2

- Spinach 5 c packed

- Coconut oil 1 T

- Carrot 1 halved

- White onion .5 sliced thin

- Shitake mushrooms 5 oz. sliced

- Zucchini 1 sliced

- Sesame oil 1 T

- Honey 2 tsp.

- Soy sauce 2 T

1.Fill a small pot with water before placing it on the stove over a burner turned to high heat.

2.While waiting for the pot to boil, combine the soy sauce, honey, sesame oil in a small bowl, whisk well and set to one side.

3.After the water, boils add in the spinach and cook until it begins to wilt. Remove it from the water with the help of a slotted spoon and squeeze out any excess water.

4.Add the oil to the skillet before placing it on the stove over a burner turned to medium heat.

5.Add in the onion, carrot and shitake mushrooms before allowing them to cook approximately 5 minutes.

6.Add in the zoodles and toss approximately 2 minutes. Add the results to a colander and toss to remove excess moisture.

7.Return the zoodles to the skillet, add in the spinach and top with the sauce. Toss for approximately 60 seconds.

Braised Collards with Dry Wine

Prep Time: 10 minutes | **Serve:** 4

- 1 pound Collards, torn into pieces

- 1 ½ tablespoons sesame oil

- 1 teaspoon ginger-garlic paste

- Sea salt and ground black pepper, to taste 1/2 teaspoon mustard seeds 1/2 teaspoon fennel seeds

- 3/4 cup water

- 1/4 cup dry red wine

1.Simply throw all of the above ingredients into your Instant Pot.

2.Secure the lid. Choose "Manual" mode and High pressure; cook for 2 minutes. Once cooking is complete, use a quick pressure release; carefully remove the lid.

3.Ladle into individual bowls and serve warm. Bon appétit!

Nutrition: 91 Calories; 9g Fat; 7g Total Carbs; 7g, Protein; 1g Sugars

Curry Cauliflower

Prep Time: 10 minutes | **Serve:** 4

- 2 tablespoons grapeseed oil

- ½ cup scallions, chopped

- 2 cloves garlic, pressed

- 1 tablespoon garam masala

- 1 teaspoon curry powder

- 1 red chili pepper, minced

- ½ teaspoon ground cumin

- Sea salt and ground black pepper, to taste 1 tablespoon fresh coriander, chopped 1 teaspoon ajwain

- 2 tomatoes, puréed

- 1 pound cauliflower, broken into florets 1/2 cup water

- ½ cup almond yogurt

1.Press the "Sauté" button to heat your Instant Pot. Now, heat the oil and sauté the scallions for 1 minute.

2.Add garlic and continue to cook an additional 30 seconds or until aromatic.

3.Add garam masala, curry powder, chili pepper, cumin, salt, black pepper, coriander, ajwain, tomatoes, cauliflower, and water.

4.Secure the lid. Choose "Manual" mode and High pressure; cook for 3 minutes. Once cooking is complete, use a quick pressure release; carefully remove the lid.

5.Pour in the almond yogurt, stir well and serve warm.

Nutrition: 101 Calories; 2g Fat; 6g Total Carbs; 3g, Protein; 36g Sugars

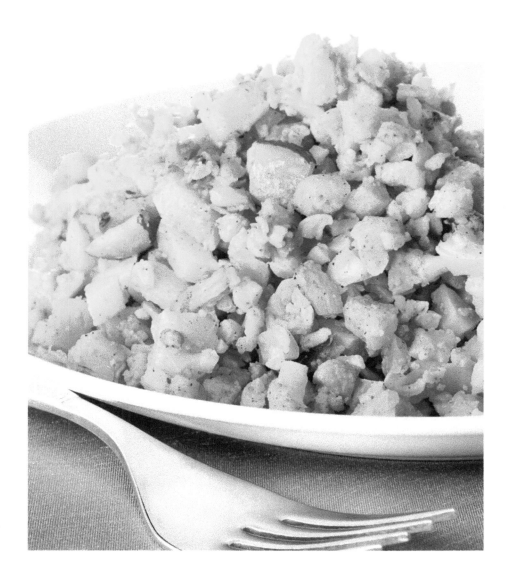

Gruel with Coconut and Seeds

Prep Time: 10 minutes | **Serve:** 4

- 4 tablespoons shredded coconut, unsweetened
- 2 tablespoons pumpkin seeds
- 2 tablespoons flaxseed
- ½ cup almonds, chopped
- ½ teaspoon grated nutmeg
- ¼ teaspoon ground cloves
- 1 teaspoon ground cinnamon
- Himalayan salt, to taste
- 1 cup boiling water

1.Add all ingredients to the Instant Pot.

2.Secure the lid. Choose "Manual" mode and High

pressure; cook for 5 minutes. Once cooking is complete,

use a quick pressure release; carefully remove the lid.

3.Serve garnished with some extra slivered almonds if

desired.

Nutrition: 116 Calories; 15g Fat; 4g Total Carbs; 7g,

Protein; 8g Sugars

Breakfast Raspberry and Walnut Cereal

Prep Time: 2 hours 10 minutes | **Serve:** 4

- 3/4 cup walnuts, soaked overnight and chopped
- Himalayan salt, to taste
- ¾ cup water
- 2 tablespoons coconut oil
- 1 tablespoon sunflower seeds
- ½ cup dried raspberries
- ½ teaspoon vanilla paste
- ¼ teaspoon star anise, ground
- ¼ teaspoon grated nutmeg
- ½ teaspoon ground cinnamon

1.Add all ingredients to your Instant Pot.

2.Secure the lid. Choose "Slow Cook" mode and High pressure; cook for 2 hours. Once cooking is complete, use a quick pressure release; carefully remove the lid.

3.Spoon into individual bowls and serve warm. Bon appétit!

Nutrition: 199 Calories; 17g Fat; 7g Total Carbs; 1g, Protein; 9g Sugars

Keto Lasagna with Cashew-Spinach Sour Cream

Prep Time: 1 hour 20 minutes | **Serve:** 4

Herbed Tomato Sauce:

- 2 teaspoons olive oil

- ½ cup green onions, chopped

- 1 garlic clove, minced

- 2 ripe tomatoes, crushed

- ½ cup water

- 1/2 teaspoon dried rosemary

- 1/2 teaspoon dried basil

- Sea salt and ground black pepper, to taste 1/2 teaspoon cayenne pepper

Cashew-Spinach Sour Cream:

- ½ cup cashews, soaked

- 1 cup water

- 1 cup spinach leaves, torn into pieces

- 2 garlic cloves

- Sea salt and ground black pepper, to taste

Zoodles:

- 4 zucchinis, sliced

- 1 tablespoon salt

- 1/2 teaspoon dried dill

- 2 tablespoons olive oil

1.Press the "Sauté" button to heat your Instant Pot. Now, heat 2 teaspoons of olive oil and sauté the green onions and garlic approximately 2 minutes.

2.Add the tomatoes, water, rosemary, basil, salt, black pepper, and cayenne pepper. Cook until thoroughly heated or approximately 5 minutes.

3.Mix cashews, water, spinach, garlic, salt, and black pepper until everything is well incorporated; reserve.

4.Slice zucchinis and add 1 tablespoon of salt. Let it sit for 30 minutes; drain your zucchinis and season them with dried dill. Now, place 1/2 of zucchini slices on the bottom of a lightly greased casserole dish.

5.Drizzle with 1 tablespoon of olive oil.

6.Add the prepared tomato sauce. Add the remaining 1/2 zucchini slices. Drizzle with 1 tablespoon of olive oil. Top with Cashew-Spinach Sour Cream.

7.Cover the casserole dish with a piece of foil.

8.Secure the lid. Choose "Bean/Chili" mode and High pressure; cook for 25 minutes. Once cooking is complete, use a quick pressure release; carefully remove the lid.

9.Allow this lasagna to cool for 10 to 15 minutes until slicing and serving. Serve warm.

Nutrition: 170 Calories; 17g Fat; 6g Total Carbs; 5g, Protein; 7g Sugars

Yummy Family Tacos

Prep Time: 45 minutes | **Serve:** 4

- 1 cup water

- 1 teaspoon ginger-garlic paste

- 2 tablespoons tamari sauce

- 1/4 cup dry white wine

Salt and pepper, to taste

- ½ teaspoon turmeric powder

- 1 teaspoon hot sauce

- 14 ounces extra-firm tofu, pressed and cubed

- 2 tablespoons olive oil

- 1 cup cherry tomatoes, halved

- 1 tablespoon Dijon mustard

- 1 bell pepper, seeded and chopped

- 1 red chili pepper, seeded and minced

Vegan Keto Tortillas:

- 2 tablespoons psyllium husks

- 1 cup almond flour

- ¼ teaspoon baking soda

- ¼ teaspoon baking powder

- Sea salt, to taste

- 2 tablespoons coconut oil, softened

- Hot water, as needed

1.In a mixing dish, combine water, ginger-garlic paste, tamari sauce, wine, salt, pepper, turmeric powder, and hot sauce; add tofu and let it marinate for 30 minutes.

2.Press the "Sauté" button to heat your Instant Pot. Heat the olive oil and brown tofu for 1 to 2 minutes per side.

3.Add the marinade. Secure the lid. Choose "Manual" mode and High pressure; cook for 6 minutes. Once cooking is complete, use a quick pressure release; carefully remove the lid.

4.Thoroughly combine dry ingredients for vegan keto tortillas; add coconut oil and mix again. Now, pour in hot water to form a dough.

5.Divide dough into 4 balls. Flatten each ball into tortilla shapes.

6.Afterwards, grill your tortillas at 350 degrees F until slightly browned on each side.

7.Assemble your tortillas with the prepared tofu, cherry tomatoes, mustard, bell pepper and chili pepper.

Nutrition: 251 Calories; 22g Fat; 7g Total Carbs; 13g, Protein; 1g Sugars

Medley with Spinach and Cauliflower

Prep Time: 10 minutes | **Serve:** 4

- 1 pound cauliflower, broken into florets
- 2 tablespoons olive oil
- 2 garlic cloves, crushed
- 1 yellow onion, peeled and chopped
- 1 celery stalk, chopped
- 1 red bell pepper, seeded and chopped Sea salt and ground black pepper, to taste 1 teaspoon Hungarian paprika
- 1 tablespoon grated lemon zest
- 2 cups spinach, torn into pieces

1.Add cauliflower, olive oil, garlic, onion, celery, bell pepper, salt, pepper, paprika, and lemon zest to the Instant Pot.

2.Secure the lid. Choose "Manual" mode and High pressure; cook for 3 minutes. Once cooking is complete, use a quick pressure release; carefully remove the lid.

3.Add spinach and put the lid on the Instant Pot. Let it sit in the residual heat until wilted.

Nutrition: 124 Calories; 5g Fat; 7g Total Carbs; 9g, Protein; 4g Sugars

Breakfast Granola with a Twist

Prep Time: 2 hours 35 minutes | **Serve:** 6

- 1 cup almonds

- 1 cup walnuts

- 2 ounces shredded coconut, unsweetened 1/4 cup sunflower seeds 1/4 cup pumpkin seeds

- 1 teaspoon vanilla paste

- 1/2 teaspoon ground cinnamon

- A pinch of kosher salt

- 1/4 teaspoon star anise, ground

- 2 tablespoons dark rum

1.Place all ingredients in your Instant Pot.

2.Secure the lid. Choose "Slow Cook" mode and High pressure; cook for 2 hours 30 minutes. Once cooking is complete, use a quick pressure release; carefully remove the lid.

3.Spoon into individual bowls and serve warm. Bon appétit!

Nutrition: 166 Calories; 12g Fat; 4g Total Carbs; 8g, Protein; 9g Sugars

Keto "Tagliatelle" with Almond Butter

Prep Time: 10 minutes | **Serve:** 4

- 2 tablespoons coconut oil

- 1 yellow onion, chopped

- 2 zucchini, julienned

- 1 cup Chinese cabbage, shredded

- 2 garlic cloves, minced

- 2 tablespoons almond butter

- Sea salt and freshly ground black pepper, to taste 1 teaspoon cayenne pepper

1.Press the "Sauté" button to heat your Instant Pot. Heat the coconut oil and sweat the onion for 2 minutes.

2.Add the other ingredients.

3.Secure the lid. Choose "Manual" mode and High

pressure; cook for 2 minutes. Once cooking is complete,

use a quick pressure release; carefully remove the lid.

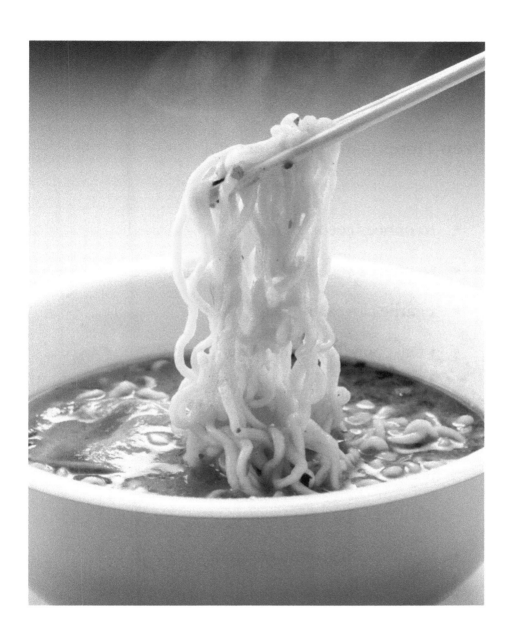

Holiday One-Pot-Wonder

Prep Time: 15 minutes | **Serve:** 4

- 10 ounces coconut milk

- 10 ounces vegetable stock

- 1 garlic cloves, minced

- 1 teaspoon fresh ginger root, grated

- 4 tablespoons almond butter

- Sea salt and ground black pepper, to taste 1/2 teaspoon turmeric powder A pinch of grated nutmeg

- ½ teaspoon ground coriander

- 10 ounces pumpkin, cubed

- 1/3 cup leek, white part only, finely sliced

1.Place the milk, stock, garlic, ginger, almond butter, salt, black pepper, turmeric powder, nutmeg, coriander, and pumpkin in your Instant Pot.

2.Secure the lid. Choose "Manual" mode and High pressure; cook for 10 minutes. Once cooking is complete, use a natural pressure release; carefully remove the lid.

3.Now, blend your soup with a stick blender. Ladle your soup into serving bowls and top with leeks. Bon appétit!

Nutrition: 157 Calories; 13g Fat; 4g Total Carbs; 4g, Protein; 7g Sugars

Vegan Keto Soup

Prep Time: 15 minutes | **Serve:** 4

- 2 tablespoons olive oil

- 1 shallot, chopped

- 1 celery, diced

- 3 ripe medium-sized tomatoes, puréed

- 4 cups roasted vegetable stock

- 1 teaspoon granulated garlic

- ½ teaspoon rosemary

- ½ teaspoon lemon thyme

- Himalayan salt and ground white pepper, to taste

- 1 bay leaf

- 4-5 whole cloves

- ½ cup almond milk, unsweetened

- 2 heaping tablespoons fresh parsley, roughly chopped

1.Press the "Sauté" button to heat your Instant Pot. Heat the olive oil and sauté the shallot and celery until softened.

2.Now, add tomatoes, stock, garlic, rosemary, lemon thyme, salt, black pepper, bay leaf, cloves, and milk; stir to combine well.

3.Secure the lid. Choose "Manual" mode and High pressure; cook for 8 minutes. Once cooking is complete, use a natural pressure release; carefully remove the lid.

4.Ladle into individual bowls and top each serving with fresh parsley.

Nutrition: 136 Calories; 8g Fat; 8g Total Carbs; 2g, Protein; 3g Sugars

Creamy Chowder with Asparagus and Mushroom

Prep Time: 15 minutes | **Serve:** 4

- 2 tablespoons coconut oil

- ½ cup shallots, chopped

- 2 cloves garlic, minced

- 1 pound asparagus, washed, trimmed and chopped

- 4 ounces button mushrooms, sliced

- 4 cups vegetable broth

- 2 tablespoons balsamic vinegar

- Himalayan salt, to taste

- ¼ teaspoon ground black pepper

- ¼ teaspoon paprika

- ¼ cup vegan sour cream

1.Press the "Sauté" button to heat your Instant Pot. Heat the oil and cook the shallots and garlic for 2 to 3 minutes.

2.Add the remaining ingredients, except for sour cream, to the Instant Pot.

3.Secure the lid. Choose "Manual" mode and High pressure; cook for 4 minutes. Once cooking is complete, use a quick pressure release; carefully remove the lid.

4.Spoon into four soup bowls; add a dollop of sour cream to each serving and serve immediately. Bon appétit!

Nutrition: 171 Calories; 17g Fat; 2g Total Carbs; 7g, Protein; 4g Sugars

Mushroom Delight with Barbecue Sauce

Prep Time: 10 minutes | **Serve:** 4

- 1 pound brown mushrooms

Barbecue sauce:

- 10 ounces tomato paste
- 1 cup water
- Sea salt and ground black pepper, to taste 1/2 teaspoon porcini powder 1 teaspoon shallot powder
- 1 teaspoon garlic powder
- 1 teaspoon mustard seeds
- ½ teaspoon fennel seeds
- 2 tablespoons lime juice

- 1 tablespoon coconut aminos

- A few drops liquid Stevia

- 1 teaspoon liquid smoke

1.Clean and slice the mushrooms; set them aside.

2.Add the remaining ingredients to your Instant Pot

andstir to combine; stir in the mushrooms.

3.Secure the lid. Choose "Manual" mode and High

pressure; cook for 4 minutes. Once cooking is complete,

use a natural pressure release; carefully remove the lid.

Serve warm.

Mediterranean Zoodles with Avocado

Prep Time: 10 minutes | **Serve:** 2

- 2 tablespoon olive oil

- 2 tomatoes, chopped

- 1 teaspoon garlic, smashed

- 1 tablespoon fresh rosemary, chopped 1/2 cup fresh parsley, roughly chopped 1/2 cup water

- 3 tablespoons almonds, ground

- 1 tablespoon apple cider vinegar

- 2 zucchinis, spiralized

- ½ avocado, pitted and sliced

- Salt and ground black pepper, to taste

1.Add olive oil, tomatoes, garlic, rosemary, parsley, water, ground almonds, and apple cider vinegar to your Instant Pot.

2.Secure the lid. Choose "Manual" mode and High pressure; cook for 5 minutes. Once cooking is complete, use a natural pressure release; carefully remove the lid.

3.Divide zoodles between two serving plates. Spoon the sauce over each serving. Top with avocado slices.

4.Season with salt and black pepper to taste. Bon appétit!

Chinese Vegan Stew

Prep Time: 20 minutes | **Serve:** 4

- 2 tablespoons sesame oil

- 1 red onion, chopped

- 1 teaspoon ginger-garlic paste

- 1 celery stalk, sliced

- 1 carrot, sliced

- 3 cups brown mushrooms, sliced

- 2 ripe Roma tomatoes, puréed

- 1 cup vegetable broth, preferably homemade

- 1 (12-ounce) bottle amber beer

- 2 bay leaves

- ½ teaspoon caraway seeds

- ¼ teaspoon cumin seeds

- ½ teaspoon fenugreek seeds

- Sea salt and ground black pepper, to taste 1 teaspoon Hungarian hot paprika 1 tablespoon soy sauce

1.Press the "Sauté" button to heat your Instant Pot. Heat the sesame oil and cook the onions for 2 to 3 minutes or until tender and translucent.

2.Now, add ginger-garlic paste, celery, carrot and mushrooms; continue to cook for a further 2 minutes or until fragrant.

3.Add the remaining ingredients, except for soy sauce.

4.Secure the lid. Choose "Manual" mode and High pressure; cook for 10 minutes. Once cooking is complete, use a quick pressure release; carefully remove the lid.

5.Ladle into individual bowls, add a few drizzles of soy sauce and serve warm. Bon appétit!

Nutrition: 136 Calories; 3g Fat; 4g Total Carbs; 6g,

Protein; 5g Sugars

Chunky Autumn Chowder

Prep Time: 10 minutes | **Serve:** 4

- 1 ½ tablespoons olive oil

- 1 leek, chopped

- 2 cloves garlic, smashed

- 1 parsnip, chopped

- 1 celery stalk, chopped

- 4 cups water

- 2 bouillon cubes

- ½ pound green cabbage, shredded

- 1 zucchini, sliced

- 2 bay leaves

- ½ teaspoon ground cumin

- ½ teaspoon turmeric powder

- 1 teaspoon dried basil

- Kosher salt and ground black pepper, to taste 6 ounces Swiss chard

1.Press the "Sauté" button to heat your Instant Pot. Heat the olive oil and cook the leek for 2 to 3 minutes or until it is softened.

2.Add the other ingredients, except forSwiss chard, to the Instant Pot; stir to combine well.

3.Secure the lid. Choose "Manual" mode and High pressure; cook for 3 minutes. Once cooking is complete, use a quick pressure release; carefully remove the lid.

4.Add Swiss chard and cover with the lid. Allow it to sit in the residual heat until it is wilted.

5.Discard bay leaves and ladle into soup bowls.

Nutrition: 99 Calories; 5g Fat; 2g Total Carbs; 2g,

Protein; 4g Sugars

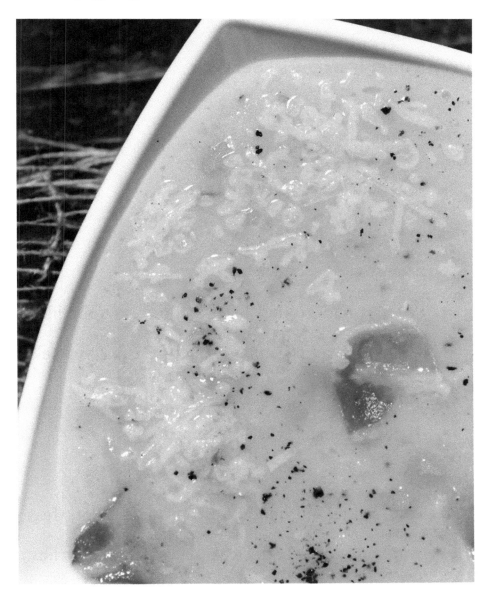

Chowder with Zucchini and Leek

Prep Time: 15 minutes | **Serve:** 4

- 2 tablespoons coconut oil

- 1 medium-sized leek, thinly sliced

- 1 zucchini, chopped

- 2 garlic cloves, crushed

- Sea salt and ground black pepper, to your liking 1/2 teaspoon cayenne pepper 4 cups vegetable stock

- ¼ cup coriander leaves, chopped

1.Press the "Sauté" button to heat your Instant Pot. Heat the coconut oil and sauté the leeks, zucchini, and garlic.

2.Next, stir in the salt, black pepper, cayenne pepper, and stock.

3.Secure the lid. Choose "Manual" mode and High pressure; cook for 8 minutes. Once cooking is complete, use a natural pressure release; carefully remove the lid.

4.Serve warm garnished with coriander leaves.

Nutrition: 90 Calories; 4g Fat; 9g Total Carbs; 2g, Protein; 5g Sugars

Baked Lamb Stew

Prep Time: 15 min | **Cook Time:** 1 h 10 min | **Serve:** 4

For Lamb Marinade:

- 3 large garlic cloves, minced

- 1 tablespoon fresh ginger, minced

- 1 lemongrass stalk, minced

- 2 tablespoons coconut aminos

- 2 tablespoons tapioca starch

- Salt and freshly ground black pepper, to taste 2-3 pound boneless lamb shoulder, trimmed and cubed into 2-inch pieces

For Stew:

- 2 tablespoons coconut oil

- 4 shallots, minced

- 2 Thai chilies, minced

- 2 tablespoons tomato paste

- 4 large tomatoes, chopped

- 4 carrots, peeled and chopped

- 1 butternut squash, peeled and cubed

- 2 stars anise

- 1 cinnamon stick

- 1 teaspoon Chinese 5-spice powder

- 2½ cups hot beef broth

1.For lamb marinade in a large glass bowl, add all ingredients and mix well.

2.Cover and refrigerate to marinate for about 2-8 hours.

3.Preheat the oven to 325 degrees F.

4.In an oven proof casserole dish, heat oil on medium-high heat.

5.Add lamb and cook for about 4-5 minutes.

6.Reduce the heat to medium.

7.Add shallots and chilies and cook for about 2-3 minutes.

8.Stir in tomato paste and tomatoes and cook for about 1-2 minutes.

9.Add remaining ingredients and stir to combine well.

10.Cover the casserole dish and immediately, transfer into oven.

11.Bake for about 1 hour or till desired doneness.

Haddock & Potato Stew

Prep Time: 15 min | **Cook Time:** 13 min | **Serve:** 4

- 2 large Yukon Gold potatoes, sliced into ¼-inch size
- 1 tbsp olive oil
- 1 (2-inch) piece fresh ginger, chopped finely
- 1 (16-ounce) can whole tomatoes, crushed ½ cup water
- 1 cup clam juice
- ¼ teaspoon red pepper flakes, crushed
- Salt, to taste
- 1½ pound boneless haddock, cut into 2inch pieces
  2 tablespoons fresh parsley, chopped

Arrange a steamer basket in a large pan of water and bring to a boil.

1.Place the potatoes in steamer basket and cook, covered for about 8 minutes.

2.Meanwhile in a pan, heat oil on medium heat.

3.Add ginger and sauté for about 1 minute.

4.Add tomatoes and cook, stirring continuously for about 2 minutes.

5.Add water, clam juice, red pepper flakes and bring to a boil.

6.Simmer for about 5 minutes, stirring occasionally.

7.Gently, stir in haddock pieces and simmer, covered for about 5 minutes or till desired doneness.

8.In serving bowls, divide potatoes and top with haddock mixture.

9.Garnish with parsley and serve.

Adzuki Beans & Carrot Stew

Prep Time: 15 min | **Cook Time:** 1 h 18 min | **Serve:** 4

- 2 tablespoons olive oil

- 1 large yellow onion, chopped

- 5 (½-inch) fresh ginger slices

- Salt, to taste

- 3 cups water

- 1 cup dried adzuki beans, soaked for overnight, rinsed and drained

- 4 large carrots, peeled and sliced into ¾-inch pieces

- 2 tablespoons brown rice vinegar

- 3 tablespoons tamari

- ½ cup fresh parsley, minced

1.In a large pan, heat oil on medium heat.

2.Add onion, ginger and salt and sauté for about 2-3 minutes.

3.Add water and beans and bring to a boil.

4.Reduce the heat to low and simmer, covered for about 45 minutes.

5.Arrange carrot slices over beans and simmer, covered for about 20-30 minutes.

6.Stir in vinegar and tamari and remove from heat.

7.Discard te ginger slices before serving.

8.Serve hot with garnishing of parsley.

Black-Eyed Beans Stew

Prep Time: 15 m | **Cook Time:** 2 h 20 m | **Serve:** 4-5

- 2 cups dried black eyed beans, soaked for overnight, rinsed and drained
- 2 medium onions, chopped and divided
- 1 (4-inch) piece fresh ginger chopped
- 4 garlic cloves, chopped
- ¼ cup olive oil
- 2 scotch bonnet peppers
- 2 (14-ounce) cans plum tomatoes
- ½-¾ cup water
- 1 vegetable bouillon cube
- Salt, to taste

1.In a large pan of boiling water, add beans and cook, covered for about 60-90 minutes or till bens become soft.

2.In a blender, add 1 onion, ginger and garlic and pulse till a puree forms.

3.In a large pan, heat oil on medium heat.

4.Add onion and sauté for about 2-5 minutes.

5.Stir in 5 tablespoons of onion puree and cook for about 5 minutes.

6.Meanwhile in blender, add bonnet peppers and tomatoes and pulse till smooth.

7.Add tomato mixture and stir to combine.

8.Reduce the heat to low and simmer, covered for about 30 minutes, stirring occasionally.

9.Stir in beans, cube and salt and simmer for about 10 minutes.

Creamy Chickpeas Stew

Prep Time: 15 min | **Cook Time:** 56 min | **Serve:** 4-6

- ¼ cup coconut oil

- 1 medium yellow onion, chopped

- 2 teaspoons fresh ginger, chopped finely

- 2 minced garlic cloves

- 1 teaspoon ground cumin

- 1 teaspoon ground coriander

- ¾ teaspoon ground turmeric

- ¼ teaspoon yellow mustard seeds

- ¼ tsp cayenne pepper

- 1 (19-ounce) can chickpeas, rinsed and drained

- 2 large sweet potatoes, peeled and cubed into 1-inch size

- 1 pound fresh kale, trimmed and chopped

- 5 cups vegetable broth

- Salt, to taste

- 1 cup coconut milk

- ¼ cup red bell pepper, seeded and julienned 2 tablespoons fresh cilantro, chopped

1.In a large pan, heat oil on medium heat.

2.Add onion and sauté for about 3 minutes.

3.Add ginger and garlic and sauté for about 2 minutes.

4.Add spices and sauté for about 1 minute.

5.Add chickpeas, sweet potato, kale and broth and bring to a boil on medium-high heat.

6.Reduce the heat to medium-low and simmer, covered for about 35 minutes.

7.Stir in coconut milk and simmer for about 15 minutes or till desired thickness of stew.

8.Serve hot with garnishing of bell pepper and cilantro.

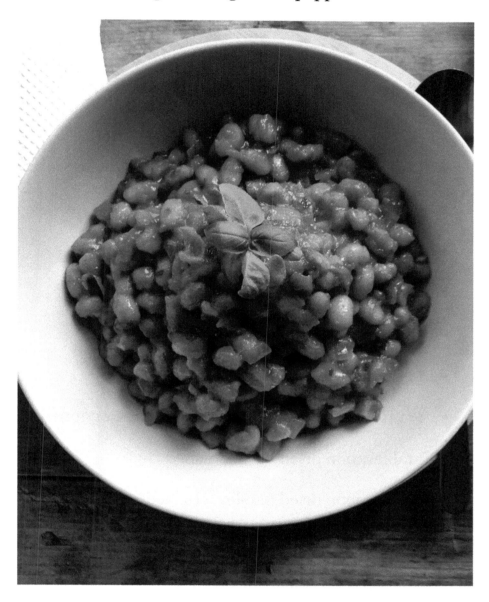

Lentil Stew

Prep Time: 15 min | **Cook Time:** 50 min | **Serve:** 4

- 1 cup dry lentils, rinsed and drained

- 1 cup potato, peeled and chopped

- ½ cup celery, chopped

- ½ cup carrot, peeled and chopped

- ½ cup onion, chopped

- 1 garlic clove, minced

- 1 (14½-ounce) peeled Italian tomatoes, chopped

- 1 tablespoon dried basil, crushed

- 1 tablespoon dried parsley, crushed

- Freshly ground black pepper, to taste

- 3½ cups chicken broth

1.In a large pan, add all ingredients and stir to combine.

2.Bring to a boil on high heat.

3.Reduce the heat to low and simmer, covered for about 45-50 minutes, stirring occasionally.

Nutrition: Calories: 261, Fat: 1g, Sat Fat: 5g, Carbohydrates: 43g, Fiber: 18g, Sugar: 2g, Protein: 19g, Sodium: 678mg

Lentil & Quinoa Stew

Prep Time: 15 min | **Cook Time:** 34 min | **Serve:** 4-6

- 1 tablespoon coconut oil

- 3 carrots, peeled and chopped

- 3 celery stalks, chopped

- 1 yellow onion, chopped

- 4 garlic cloves, minced

- 1 (26½-ounce) can chopped tomatoes

- 1 cup red lentils, rinsed and drained

- ½ cup quinoa

- 1½ teaspoons ground cumin

- ½ teaspoon ground turmeric

- ½ teaspoon ground ginger

- Salt, to taste

- 5 cups water

- 2 cups fresh kale, chopped

1.In a large pan, heat oil on medium heat.

2.Add celery, onion and carrot and sauté for about 8 minutes.

3.Add garlic and sauté for about 1 minute.

4.Add remaining ingredients except kale and bring to a boil.

5.Reduce the heat to low and simmer, covered for about 20 minutes.

6.Stir in kale and simmer for about 4-5 minutes.

Chilled Tomato & Bell Pepper Soup

Prep Time: 25 min | **Cook Time:** 20 sec | **Serve:** 4-6

- 8 ripe Roma tomatoes
- 1 small red bell pepper, seeded and chopped roughly
- 1 small green bell pepper, seeded and chopped roughly
- 1 medium cucumber, peeled, seeded and chopped roughly
- 1 small red onion, chopped roughly
- 3 large garlic cloves, chopped
- 1 fresh long red chili, seeded and chopped roughly
- 2 teaspoons fresh orange zest, grated finely

- 1 cup fresh tomato juice

- ¾ cup olive oil

- 2-3 tablespoons fresh orange juice

- 2 tablespoons apple cider vinegar

- 1 cup chilled water

- 1 teaspoon salt

- ½ freshly ground black pepper

1.In a large pan of boiling water, add tomatoes and boil for 20 seconds or till the skin begins to crack.

2.Drain well and rinse under cold water. Then peel the skin of tomatoes. Cut the tomatoes and discard the seeds.

3.In a large food processor, add tomatoes and keep all ingredients and pulse till smooth.

4.Refrigerate to chill for about 1 hour before serving.

Chilled Peas Soup

Prep Time: 10 min | **Cook Time:** 20 sec | **Serve:** 4

- ½ tablespoons coconut oil

- 1 large shallot, minced

- 10 fresh mint leaves

- 2 cups homemade chicken broth

- 1 pound frozen baby peas

- Salt and freshly ground black pepper, to taste

1.In a medium pan, heat oil on medium-high heat.

2.Add shallots and sauté for about 1 minute.

3.Add mint and broth and bring to a boil.

4.Stir in peas and again bring to a boil.

5.Reduce the heat to medium-low. Simmer for about 4 minutes.

6.Season with salt and black pepper and remove from heat. Let it cool slightly.

7.Transfer the soup in a blender and pulse till smooth.

8.Refrigerate to chill for about 1 hour before serving.

Nutrition: Calories: 119, fat: 9g, carbohydrates: 18g, sugar: 9g, protein: 7g, fiber: 7g

Chilled Spinach & Cucumber Soup

Prep Time: 15 minutes | **Serve:** 2

- 2 medium cucumbers, peeled seeded and chopped
- 2 cups fresh spinach
- 1 small avocado, peeled, pitted and chopped ½ of jalapeño, seeded and chopped 1cup mixed fresh herbs
- 1 cup water
- 1 tablespoon fresh lime juice
- 1 tablespoon olive oil

1.In a large food processor, add all ingredients and pulse till smooth.

2.Refrigerate to chill for about 2 hours before serving.

Chilled Fruit Soup

Prep Time: 15 minutes | **Serve:** 4

For Soup:

- 2 pounds fresh strawberries, hulled and sliced ½ of medium watermelon, seeded and chopped

For Raspberry Sauce:

- 6-ounce fresh raspberries
- ¼ cup coconut milk
- 1 teaspoon fresh lemon zest, grated finely
- 1 tablespoon fresh lemon juice

1.In a bowl, add watermelon and strawberries. With a hand blender, blend till a smooth and creamy mixture forms.

2.Refrigerate to chill.

3.In a bowl, add raspberries and mash with a fork completely.

4.Add remaining ingredients and stir to combine well. Refrigerate to chill.

5.Divide the soup in serving bowls. Top with raspberry sauce and serve.

Chilled Pineapple Soup

Prep Time: 15 minutes | **Serve:** 4

- 1 under ripe pineapple, peeled, cored and chopped ½ cup cucumber, peeled, seeded and chopped finely ½ cup red bell pepper, seeded and chopped finely ¼ cup red onion, chopped finely
- 1 tablespoon fresh cilantro, chopped finely ¼ of serrano Chile, seeded and minced
- 2 tablespoons fresh lime juice
- ½ teaspoon salt

1.In a blender, add pineapple and pulse till pureed.

2.Strain the puree in a bowl.

3.Stir in remaining ingredients. Cover and chill for about 2 hours before serving.

Creamy Cauliflower Soup

Prep Time: 15 m | **Cook Time:** 22-25 m | **Serve:** 4-6

- 1 tablespoon extra-virgin olive oil

- 1 medium onion, chopped

- 4 garlic cloves, minced

- Salt, to taste

- 1 medium head cauliflower, cut into 1-inch pieces

- 4 ½-5½ cups water

- 1 avocado, peeled, pitted and chopped

- 2-3 cups mixed greens

- Freshly ground black pepper, to taste

- Fresh chopped parsley, for garnishing

1.In a large soup pan, heat oil on medium heat.

2.Add onion and sauté for about 4-5 minutes.

3.Add garlic and pinch of salt and sauté for about 2-3 minutes.

4.Stir in cauliflower and ad water. Bring to a boil on high heat.

5.Reduce the heat to low. Simmer for about 10 minutes.

6.Stir in avocado and greens and simmer for about 3 minutes.

7.Remove from heat and cool slightly.

8.In a blender, transfer the soup in batches and pulse till smooth.

9.Add the soup in the pan on medium heat. Cook for about 3-4 minutes.

10.Stir in salt and black pepper and remove from heat.

11.Serve with the garnishing of parsley.

Creamy Carrot Soup

Prep Time: 15 min | **Cook Time:** 25 min | **Serve:** 2-3

- 3 cups homemade vegetable broth

- 1½ cups fennel bulb, chopped

- 3 cups carrots, peeled and chopped

- 2 garlic cloves, minced

- 1 cup full-fat coconut milk

- Salt, to taste

- 4-ounces pancetta, chopped

- ½ cup pine nuts, toasted and chopped

1.In a large soup pan, add broth and vegetables and a boil on high heat.

2.Reduce the heat to medium-low. Simmer for about 15-20 minutes.

3.Stir in coconut milk and simmer for about 3-5 minutes. Stir in salt and remove from heat.

4.Meanwhile heat a nonstick skillet on medium-high heat.

5.Add pancetta and cook for about 8-10 minutes or till crispy.

6.Serve this soup hot with the topping of cooked pancetta and pine nuts.

Green Veggie Soup

Prep Time: 20 min | **Cook Time:** 25 min | **Serve:** 6

- 2 tablespoons ghee (clarified butter)

- 3-4 garlic cloves, minced

- 4 leeks (white part), chopped roughly

- 2 medium heads broccoli, chopped roughly ½ of small head cauliflower, chopped roughly 4 celery sticks, chopped roughly

- 8 cups homemade vegetable broth

- 2-3 cups fresh baby spinach

- 1 cup fresh parsley, chopped

- Freshly ground black pepper, to taste

- Pinch of ground nutmeg

- 1 tablespoon coconut cream

1.In a large soup pan, heat oil on medium heat.

2.Add garlic and leeks and sauté for about 4-5 minutes.

3.Add broccoli, cauliflower and celery and sauté for about 5 minutes.

4.Add broth and bring to a boil. Reduce the heat to low. Simmer for about 10-15 minutes.

5.Stir in spinach and parsley and remove from heat.

6.With an immense blender, blend till pureed. Stir in nutmeg and black pepper.

7.Top with the dollop of coconut cream and serve.

Nutrition: Calories: 108, fat: 3g, carbohydrates: 17g, protein: 7g, fiber: 6g

Chicken & Veggie Soup

Prep Time: 20 min | **Cook Time:** 28-30 m | **Serve:** 4

- 2 tablespoons coconut oil

- 1 bunch scallion, sliced thinly

- 2-inch piece fresh ginger, minced

- 4 garlic cloves, minced

- 1 cup shiitake mushrooms, sliced

- 1 large carrot, peeled and shredded

- 1 red bell pepper, seeded and chopped

- 1 jalapeño pepper, chopped

- 14-ounces coconut milk

- 4 cups chicken broth

- 1 tablespoon red bat fish sauce

- 1 pound skinless, boneless chicken breasts Fresh cilantro, as required
- 1 teaspoon fresh lime zest, grated finely
- Salt and freshly ground black pepper, to taste

1.In a large soup pan, heat oil on medium heat.

2.Add scallion, ginger and garlic and sauté for about 2-3 minutes.

3.Add mushrooms, carrot, bell pepper and jalapeño pepper and sauté for about 5 minutes.

4.Add broth, coconut milk, fish sauce and chicken and bring to a boil.

5.Reduce the heat to low. Simmer for about 15 minutes.

6.Transfer the chicken into a plate and chop into small chunks.

7.Add chopped chicken, cilantro, lime zest, salt and black pepper and simmer for 5 minutes more.

Mushroom Soup

Prep Time: 20 min | **Cook Time:** 30 min | **Serve:** 4

- ½-ounce dried porcini mushrooms

- 2 tablespoons ghee (clarified butter)

- 1 celery stalk, chopped

- 1 large leek (pale part), chopped

- 1 small sweet potato, peeled and chopped

- 15 medium crimini mushrooms, sliced roughly

- 3 garlic cloves, minced

- 1 tablespoon dried thyme, crushed

- 3 cups homemade chicken broth

- ½ teaspoon Dijon mustard

- 1 tablespoon red boat fish sauce

- 2 bay leaves

- 1 teaspoon fresh lemon zest, grated finely ½ teaspoon freshly ground black pepper 3 tablespoons almond butter
- 1 tablespoon fresh lemon juice

1.In a bowl, soak porcini mushrooms in boiling water. Keep aside for about 15-20 minutes.

2.Strain the mushrooms, reserving ½ cup of liquid. Then chop the mushrooms.

3.In a large soup pan, heat ghee on medium heat.

4.Add celery and leek and sauté for about 5-7 minutes.

5.Add sweet potato, cremini mushrooms, garlic and thyme and sauté for about 1-2 minutes.

6.Add broth, mustard, fish sauce, bay leaves, lemon zest, black pepper and cremini mushrooms with reserved liquid and bring to a boil.

7.Reduce the heat to low. Cover and simmer for about 15 minutes.

8.Uncover and simmer for 5 minutes more.

9.Stir in almond butter and lemon juice and serve hot.

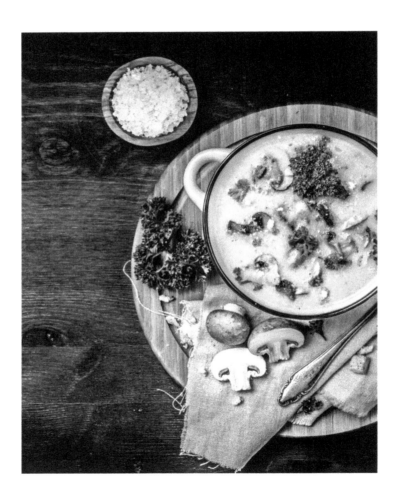

Roasted Veggies Soup

Prep Time: 20 min | **Cook Time:** 30 min | **Serve:** 4-6

- 2½ pounds zucchini, cut into 1-inch pieces ½ of yellow onion, chopped 1 leek, chopped
- 3 garlic cloves, peeled
- 2 tablespoons coconut oil, melted
- 2½ cups water
- ½ cup raw cashews, soaked for 3 hours
- Salt and freshly ground black pepper, to taste

1.Preheat the oven to 400 degrees F. Line a baking sheet with a parchment paper.

2.Arrange zucchini, onion, leek and garlic onto prepared baking sheet.

3.Roast for about 20 minutes. Remove from oven and cool slightly.

4.In a blender, add roasted veggies, water and cashews and pulse till smooth.

5.Transfer the pureed mixture in a soup pan on medium heat.

6.Simmer for about 5 minutes. Stir in salt and black pepper and remove from heat.

Chicken & Asparagus Soup

Prep Time: 20 min | **Cook Time:** 20 min | **Serve:** 8

- 1 tablespoon coconut oil

- 1 onion, chopped

- 2 cups mushrooms, sliced thinly

- 1 celery stalk, chopped

- 2 cups grass-fed boneless chicken, chopped

- 15-20 fresh asparagus spears, trimmed and chopped

- 6-8 cups homemade chicken broth

- 14-ounce coconut milk

- 2 cups fresh spinach, chopped

- Salt and freshly ground black pepper, to taste

1.In a large soup pan, heat oil on medium heat.

2.Add onion, mushrooms and celery and sauté for about 5 minutes.

3.Add chicken, asparagus and broth and bring to a boil.

4.Reduce the heat to low. Simmer for about 10 minutes.

5.Stir in coconut milk and spinach and bring to a boil on high heat.

6.Reduce the heat to low. Simmer for about 3-4 minutes.

7.Stir in salt and black pepper and remove from heat.

Shrimp & Snow Peas Soup

Prep Time: 15 min | **Cook Time:** 8-10 min | **Serve:** 8

- 4 teaspoons coconut oil

- 4 medium scallions (white and green part), sliced thinly

- 2-inch piece fresh ginger root, sliced thinly

- 8 cups homemade chicken broth

- ¼ teaspoon red boat fish sauce

- ¼ cup coconut aminos

- 1/8 teaspoon freshly ground white pepper 1 pound shrimp, peeled and deveined

- 1 (5-ounce) can sliced bamboo shoots, drained ½ pound snow peas, cleaned

- 1 tablespoon sesame oil, toasted

1.In a large soup pan, heat oil on medium heat.

2.Add white part of scallion and ginger and sauté for about 2 minutes.

3.Add broth, fish sauce, coconut aminos and white pepper and bring to a boil.

4.Stir in shrimp, bamboo shoots and snow peas.

5.Reduce the heat to low. Simmer for about 2-3 minutes.

6.Stir in sesame oil and green part of scallion and remove from heat.

Zucchini & Squash Soup

Prep Time: 15 min | **Cook Time:** 12-15 min | **Serve:** 4

- 2 tablespoons coconut oil

- 1 small onion, chopped

- 3 garlic cloves, minced

- 1 teaspoon ground cumin

- 1½ pounds yellow squash, chopped

- 3 cups zucchini, chopped

- 2 tablespoons jalapeño peppers, chopped finely

- 4 cups homemade vegetable broth

- 1 cup coconut milk

- 3 tablespoons fresh lemon juice

- ¼ cup fresh cilantro, chopped

- 2 tablespoons nutritional yeast

- Avocado slices, for garnishing

1.In a large soup pan, heat oil on medium heat.

2.Add onion and sauté for about 4-5 minutes.

3.Add garlic and cumin and sauté for about 1 minute.

4.Add squash and zucchini and sauté for about 3-4 minutes.

5.Add jalapeño peppers and broth and bring to a boil. Immediately, turn off the heat.

6.Keep, covered for about 10 minutes.

7.Stir in coconut milk, lemon juice, cilantro and nutritional yeast and again bring to a boil.

8.Serve hot with the topping of avocado slices.

Spicy Leek Soup With Poached Eggs

Prep Time: 15 min | **Cook Time:** 10 min | **Serve:** 6-8

- 2 tablespoons coconut oil
- 1 large leek, sliced
- 4 carrots, peeled and sliced
- 6 garlic cloves, minced
- 6-8 cups chicken broth
- ¾ teaspoon dried oregano, crushed
- ½ teaspoon paprika
- Pinch of red pepper flakes, crushed
- 2 teaspoons unrefined salt
- 6-8 organic eggs

1.In a large soup pan, heat oil on medium heat.

2.Add leeks and sauté for about 3-4 minutes.

3.Add carrots and cook for about 4-5 minutes.

4.Add garlic and sauté for about 1 minute.

5.Add broth, oregano and spices and bring to a boil.
Reduce the heat to low.

6.Simmer for about 10 minutes.

7.Meanwhile in a frying pan, add 1-2-inch water and
bring to a gentle simmer. Stir in some salt.

8.Carefully, crack eggs in pan and cook for about 3-4
minutes on medium-low heat.

9.With a slotted spoon, place 1 egg in each bowl.

10. Divide the soup in bowls evenly and serve.

Parmesan Kale

Prep Time: 5 min | **Cook Time:** 20 min | **Serve:** 4

- 4 cups kale, roughly chopped

- 2 oz Parmesan, grated

- 1 tablespoon olive oil

1.Put the kale in the tray and flatten it well.

2.Then sprinkle the kale with olive oil and Parmesan.

3.Cook the kale at 350F for 20 minutes.

Nutrition: 109 calories, 6.6g protein, 7.5g carbohydrates, 6.5g fat, 1g fiber, 10mg cholesterol, 161mg sodium, 329mg potassium

Curry Tofu

Prep Time: 20 min | **Cook Time:** 5 min | **Serve:** 4

- 1-pound tofu, cubed

- 1 teaspoon curry powder

- 1 tablespoon olive oil

- ½ cup coconut cream

- 1 teaspoon lemon zest, grated

1.In the mixing bowl, mix curry powder with olive oil, coconut cream, and lemon zest.

2.Then add tofu and mix well.

3.Leave the mixture for 10 minutes to marinate.

4.Then preheat the skillet well.

5.Add tofu and cook it for 2 minutes per side.

Nutrition: 180 calories, 10.1g protein, 4g carbohydrates, 15.5g fat, 1.9g fiber, 0mg cholesterol, 18mg sodium, 256mg potassium

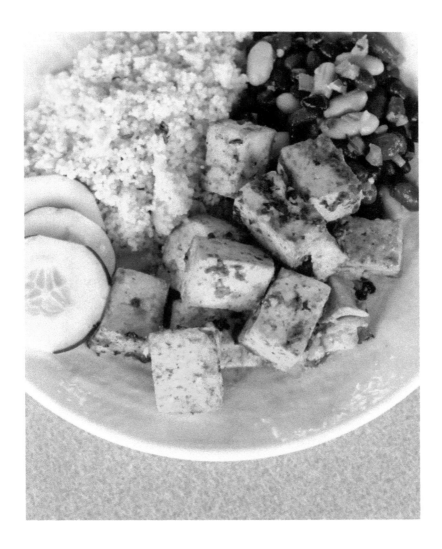

Cumin Zucchini Rings

Prep Time: 10 min | **Cook Time:** 15 min | **Serve:** 5

- 3 zucchinis, sliced
- 1 tablespoon cumin seeds
- 1 tablespoon olive oil
- ¼ teaspoon cayenne pepper

1.Line the baking tray with baking paper.

2.Put the zucchini slices inside the baking tray in one layer.

3.Then sprinkle them with cumin seeds, olive oil, and cayenne pepper.

4.Bake the zucchini rings for 15 minutes at 360F.

Nutrition: 48 calories, 1.6g protein, 4.5g carbohydrates, 3.3g fat, 1.4g fiber, 0mg cholesterol, 14mg sodium, 331mg potassium

Chickpeas Spread

Prep Time: 10 min | **Cook Time:** 0 min | **Serve:** 3

- 1 cup chickpeas, cooked

- 1 tablespoon tahini paste

- 2 tablespoons lemon juice

- ¼ cup olive oil

1.Put all ingredients in the blender.

2.Blend the mixture until smooth.

3.Transfer it in the serving bowl.

Nutrition: 419 calories, 13.8g protein, 41.7g carbohydrates, 23.6g fat, 12.1g fiber, 0mg cholesterol, 24mg sodium, 617mg potassium

Mushroom Caps

Prep Time: 10 min | **Cook Time:** 20 min | **Serve:** 5

- 5 Portobello mushrooms (caps)

- 3 oz tofu, shredded

- ½ teaspoon curry paste

- 2 tablespoons coconut cream

- 1 teaspoon olive oil

1.In the mixing bowl, mix curry powder with coconut cream, olive oil, and shredded tofu.

2.Then fill the mushrooms with the shredded tofu mixture and put in the tray in one layer.

3.Bake the mushrooms at 360F for 20 minutes.

Nutrition: 57 calories, 4.6g protein, 3.8g carbohydrates, 3.4g fat, 1.3g fiber, 0mg cholesterol, 3mg sodium, 341mg potassium

Ginger Baked Mango

Prep Time: 10 min | **Cook Time:** 20 min | **Serve:** 4

- 2 mangos, pitted, halved
- 1 teaspoon minced ginger
- 1 tablespoon olive oil
- ¼ teaspoon dried rosemary

1.Put the mango halves in the baking tray and sprinkle with olive oil.

2.Then sprinkle the fruit with minced ginger and dried rosemary.

3.Bake the mango at 360F for 20 minutes.

Nutrition: 133 calories, 1.4g protein, 25.5g carbohydrates, 4.2g fat, 2.8g fiber, 0mg cholesterol, 2mg sodium, 289mg potassium

Poached Green Beans

Prep Time: 10 min | **Cook Time:** 15 min | **Serve:** 4

- 1-pound green beans, trimmed

- 2 cups of water

- 1 garlic clove, diced

- 2 tablespoons olive oil

- 1 tablespoon lime juice

1.Bring the water to boil and add green beans. Boil them for 10 minutes.

2.Then remove the green beans from water and mix with garlic clove, olive oil, and lime juice.

Nutrition: 97 calories, 2.1g protein, 8.6g carbohydrates, 7.2g fat, 3.9g fiber, 0mg cholesterol, 11mg sodium, 244mg potassium

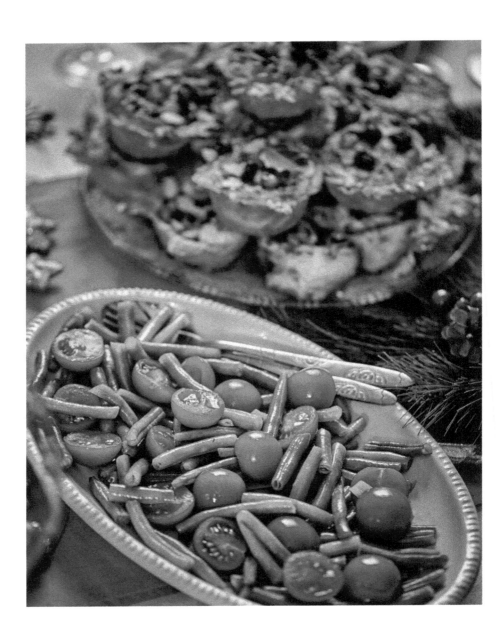

Lightning Source UK Ltd.
Milton Keynes UK
UKHW020622220722
406226UK00001B/9